BLOOD PRESS

HOW TO REDUCE HYPERTENSION

THE STEP BY STEP GUIDE ON HOW TO NATURALLY LOWER YOUR BLOOD PRESSURE IN 31 DAYS

DR. JOHN LUTZ (PH.D)

BLOOD PRESSURE

—HOW TO REDUCE—

HYPERTENSION

THE STEP BY STEP GUIDE ON HOW
TO NATURALLY LOWER YOUR BLOOD
PRESSURE IN 31 DAYS

DR. JOHN LUTZ (PH.D)

DISCLAIMER

No Personal or Medical Tips

The instructions in this book, whether provided in digital form or in hard copy is for general information purposes and nothing contained in it is, or is intended to be construed as advice. It does not report your medical, health, physical or emotional needs or cravings. It is not used instead of treatment, the attention you need medically, testing by your doctor, the medical tips you're given by your doctor, treating of already present ailments and this book is not written to give out clinical examination, or taking the place of the medical advice or tips you get from your doctor.

Before you can use or take part in this useful book, look at the suitability of it in your own personal life situations or needs. You should talk to your medical doctor before using any of the instructions that is in this book, before you embark on any treatment or taking any path that will indirectly or directly influence your health or the way you live.

COPYRIGHT

DR. JOHN LUTZ (PH.D) 2020

TABLE OF CONTENT

INTRODUCTION

Have you been tested and confirmed to have hypertension or high blood pressure? If yes! Then you're now among the half population of adults in the U.S. It is even heartbreaking that most of them (28 percent) living with this condition don't know that they have it, and that is why it is mostly referred to as the "silent killer." Your risk of having kidney failure, aneurysms, stroke, and disease of the heart will increase exponentially and it's one of the major causes of over 15% mortality rate every year in the U.S.A.

High blood pressure is not a good thing, because it can kill someone silently without that person knowing that he has it in the first place. So, when you've discovered, that you've high blood pressure, take the right step to find solution to manage or reduce it to live longer. By getting this book, you have taken the right step to improve your health, in all spheres, because this book is going to show you the secrets and steps to follow strictly in order to reduce or manage your high blood pressure.

To lower your high blood pressure, they are some things you need to do and they are some habits you need to abandon or say goodbye to. This extensive work will reveal those things to you, and also show you the ways to get rid of them in order to reduce or manage high blood pressure.

Though, high blood pressure has no respect for one's age, the major people who are mostly affected are adults. It is rare to see a teenager or a young adult been diagnosed with high blood pressure.

Everyone in this world desire to live long, but they are some ailments or health conditions which ends people's life without them even knowing, that they have it in the first place. High blood pressure is one of those conditions that can end someone's life, so it must be managed or reduced.

If you're prepared and ready to reduce your high blood pressure, then join this ride, as you glean through the pages of this book.

DR. JOHN LUTZ.
SEPTEMBER, 2020.

I WAS DIAGNOSED WITH HIGH BLOOD PRESSURE AND I FELT SAD!

When I first got diagnosed with high blood pressure, I became very sad and gloomy. In my case, it was my lifestyle that caused it, and I was aware that one day I'm going to have such issue. Nevertheless, I still continued with my lifestyle, until I got diagnosed with high blood pressure. Many habits contributed to it, but smoking of cigarette was the major contributor. I can smoke 2 packets of cigarette a day.

There was a time, I smoke 4 packets of cigarette, and I thought I was enjoying myself, but health wise; I was heading to my doom. Whenever I smoke cigarette, my body will be tensed. So, I decided to go for test and the doctor said that I have gotten high blood pressure.

At first, it sounds like a joke to me, but when I reminisced about my habits and lifestyle, I realized that I deserve what I got (high blood pressure), because countless times I was warned to quit those habits, but I did not heed to those important warnings.

Although, smoking is the key reason for my high blood pressure back then, other habits also contributed to it. Those habits and lifestyles are;

1. Excessive consumption of alcoholic drink.

2. Not taking part in exercise.

3. Bad sleep culture.

4. Over thinking.

5. Too much stress.

6. Consumption of too much salt.

''To solve a problem easily, you ought to find out the root cause of the problem.''

When I discovered that smoking, as well as other habits/lifestyle listed above – is the root of my problem (hypertension), I decided to adjust and stop those habits. At first it was hard, because I was very addicted to smoking. But with zeal and willingness to stop the addiction, I was able to quit successfully. Afterward, without meds from the doctors, I was able to lower my blood pressure.

When I stopped smoking for like a week, the difference became very clear; my blood pressure began to go down rapidly, heading to the normal/appropriate level. Smoking for me in the past, was like getting a new car. It was so dear to me, but for my health, I had to stop and it has helped me a lot.

Apart from lowering my blood pressure, some of the habit I quitted, helped me to gain weight, live a good and healthy life, sleep well, and have a good relationship with people.

I have some friends that I do advice to quit smoking, but they refused to heed to my advice. As time goes on, they were diagnosed with high blood pressure – theirs has increased exponentially. They are at a critical level – a life threatening stage. Some are regretting for not following my advice. However, some of them followed it and now their blood pressure is lowered and they are doing fine.

The same steps that I followed, that worked for me and some of my friends, is what I'm going to reveal to you in this book. Are you like my friends, who rejected my advice and end up in a critical condition (high blood pressure)? Or are you going to heed to the advice (steps and guides to lower high blood pressure) I'm going to dish out in this book, just like my other friends, who are now doing fine? The ball is in your court.

A saying goes thus; ''experience is the best teacher.'' Yes! This assertion is very true. Back then when I used to smoke, I was advised to quit the habit, but I did not heed to the advice, until I was diagnosed with high blood pressure. That is when I start making changes.

What I learnt from my experience

I learnt that, they are some habits and lifestyles that can cause us more harm, than good. The habit may be too sweet to quit or let go of, but in the long run, it may turns out to be harmful to our health and wellbeing.

I felt good smoking back then, but health wise I was slowly heading to my doom. Aside from high blood pressure and lungs damage, it can lead to other complications like poor vision, bronchitis, lung cancer, infertility, blood clotting, diabetes complications, and increased risk of blood cancer.

Some habits are not even good to be practiced. It will be good to quit a habit, if it can interfere with your health.

CHAPTER ONE

MEANING OF HIGH BLOOD PRESSURE

Now, before anything else, let's look at the meaning of high blood pressure.

MEANING: High blood pressure, which is also known as hypertension, is the situation – when your blood pressure, the force of your blood pushing against the walls of your blood vessels, is very high.

Understanding the way your circulatory system and blood pressure actually work

Your organs and tissues need the oxygenated blood that is been carried throughout the body by the circulatory system, to be able to survive and function well. There's formation of pressure, that pushes blood through a network of blood vessel which is shaped like a tube, and it includes capillaries, veins, and arteries. Two forces are key players, when it comes to this pressure and they are the reasons for blood pressure. **They are:**

1. Systolic Pressure:

These kinds of force occur as blood is being pump out of the heart into the arteries which are part of the circulatory system.

2. Diastolic Pressure

This one is formed when the heart rests between heart beats.

The above forces are each represented by numbers in a blood pressure reading.

Blood pressure can cause harm to your heart and arteries, see how below.

It all starts from your arteries and heart.

One of the major ways, high blood pressure causes damage, is by increasing the workload of the blood vessels and heart which make them to work very hard and less effective.

As time pass by, the friction and force of high blood pressure causes harm to the delicate tissues inside the arteries. In turn, LDL (bad) cholesterol forms plaque along tiny tears in the artery walls, which signal the start of atherosclerosis.

If the damage and the plaque increases exponentially, the inside of the arteries will become smaller (narrower) – and this will make the blood pressure to rise and start a vicious circle, which the end result, is harming your heart, arteries, and other parts of your body. As a result, an individual can be susceptible to other conditions like stroke, arrhythmia and heart attack.

The "silent killer" – High Blood Pressure

Blood pressure may seem like a little thing to you, however, it can cause harm or silently damage your organs and cells, which may result to it been a big threat to your life and overall health. What you need to do, to prevent this disaster is to have knowledge of your numbers and make critical, and required changes in order to manage and prevent/reduce high blood pressure.

It is a well known complication, in which the long-term force of the blood against your artery walls is high enough, that it may eventually cause health problems, like disease of the heart.

Blood pressure is determined both by the amount of blood your heart pumps and the amount of resistance to blood flow in your arteries. The narrower your arteries and the more blood your hearts pumps, the higher your blood pressure.

You can have high blood pressure (hypertension) for years, without any symptoms. In absence of symptoms, the damages it causes to your heart and blood vessels can be noticed. When high blood pressure is not controlled, it can make you vulnerable to some core health complications which include stroke and heart attack.

It takes high blood pressure many years to develop, and the effect is mostly felt by everyone eventually. However, it is easy to detect high blood pressure. As soon as you discover that you have it, is either you make some changes in your lifestyles or work with your doctor to lower or reduce it. However, this book is going to focus on making changes in your lifestyles and habits – not taking medicine or visiting a doctor. As we go further, you'll come across those habits you ought to shun and those lifestyles you need to abandon – in order to lower your blood pressure.

The Symptoms of High Blood Pressure

Generally, several people with this condition – high blood pressure do not show symptoms or signs, even when the blood pressure reaches high levels.

But some few who live with high blood pressure may have the following signs:

1. Nosebleeds or shortness of breath.

2. Headache.

Nevertheless, the above symptoms and signs are not entirely related to high blood pressure and furthermore, they don't show up, until high blood pressure has reached a dangerous and critical stage.

TYPES OF HIGH BLOOD PRESSURE

High blood pressure is of two types. There are:

1. Essential (primary) hypertension

2. Secondary hypertension

1. Essential (primary) hypertension

In some adults, there's no identifiable cause of high blood pressure. This type of high blood pressure, which is termed as primary (essential) hypertension, usually develops gradually for numerous years. It does not start just like that, but it develops for many years.

2. Secondary hypertension

Some people have high blood pressure which is mostly caused by health complications. This type of high blood pressure, which is called secondary hypertension, usually comes up in a sudden way and it cause higher blood pressure than that of primary hypertension. There are several medications and conditions that can lead to secondary hypertension, these includes:

1. Adrenal gland tumors.

2. Obstructive sleep apnea.

3. Thyroid problems.

4. A particular defects you're born with (inherited) in blood vessels.

5. Kidney problems.

6. Illegal drugs, such as cocaine and amphetamines.

7. Certain medications, like over-the-counter pain reliever, some prescription drugs, cold remedies, decongestants, and birth control pills.

Causes of High Blood Pressure / Risk Factors Associated with Hypertension and its Effects

In the world of health, in order to protect yourself from some health complication, you need to have knowledge of their causes. By having the knowledge of why those health complications do come up, you'll get to know how to live your life, in the proper way. When you get to know the causes of high blood pressure, you'll do the right thing. So below, you are going to see the causes of high blood pressure. Also, they are many risk factors associated with high blood pressure. You've to know them, to be able to handle them. You'll get to see them as you read further.

Below are the causes of high blood pressure

Tobacco usage

As earlier stated, in my real life story, about how I got diagnosed with hypertension due to my smoking habits, tobacco usage can also cause high blood pressure.

When you chew or smoke tobacco, it will instantly raise your blood pressure, aside that, the chemicals in tobacco are capable of damaging the lining of your artery walls.

When this happens, your arteries will become narrowed and your risk of getting disease of the heart will be high. Also, secondhand smoke may likely increase your risk of getting heart disease. Smoking of cigarette may seem good at first, but it will cause you more damage than good. You may get that ''calm and feel good effect'' from the onset, but the damage in the future will be tremendous. If you're an addict, try your best to quit the habit. As earlier stated, aside it raising your blood pressure, it makes you susceptible to some serious health complications. If you smoke, it will be in your best interest, to quit the habit today.

Not taking part in exercises

Someone who does not engage in exercises will likely have higher heart rates. The higher your heart rate, the harder your heart must work with each contraction and the force on your arteries will be stronger. Apart from hypertension, your risk of being overweight will be on the increase, when you don't take part in exercises.

Too much alcohol intake

If you drink alcohol excessively, with time, it may damage your heart. For women, one bottle of drink is recommended for a day and for men, it is two bottles a day. Anything more than that, it may affect your blood pressure.

It is not advisable to drink alcohol. But if you can't do without drinking alcohol, you should drink moderately. As earlier stated, for adults who are healthy, women should only drink one bottle of alcohol a day and two bottles of alcohol for men. One bottle of drink is equivalent to 12 ounces of beer, 5 ounces of wine or 1.5 ounces of 80-proof liquor. Too much alcohol intake can make you lose focus in life. Always drink in moderation. Too much intake of alcohol can lead you to have kidney disease.

Being Obese or Overweight

If your weight is much, then the more blood you'll need to supply nutrients and oxygen to your tissues. Overtime, the amount of blood circulated through your blood vessels will increase, which leads to the increase of pressure on your artery walls. Sorry to say, if you're fat or obese, you need to shed some pounds for your overall health.

Stress

Whenever you're stressed, you can experience temporal increase in blood pressure. It may become worse, if you try to relax by consuming a lot of junk food, drinking alcohol or using tobacco, because they can all leads to high blood pressure.

Age

As you depart from young age to old age, your risk of having high blood pressure will increase. High blood pressure is more common in men when they reached 64 years of age. In the same vein, women may start developing high blood pressure after crossing the age of 65.

Family history

Some families are well known as people who have high blood pressure running through their lineage. In this kind of family, everyone, from young to old has high blood pressure. It is somehow inherited. In such family, it will be hard to see an individual who does not have high blood pressure. So, don't be surprised when you see such individuals.

Dementia

If the artery is narrow, it can limit the blood flow to the brain, which in turns leads to a particular type of dementia called vascular dementia. Also, vascular dementia can be caused when a stroke interrupts blood flow to the brain.

Race

The set of people who have the highest rate of high blood pressure is the black race; it develops at an earlier age than it does in white people. Aside from hypertension, they are other health complications that are mostly common in people of African heritage. These complications are kidney failure, stroke, and heart attack.

Adding too much sodium (salt) to your diet

If you add too much salt to your diet, it will make your body to retain fluid, and when this happens, your blood pressure increases. So, try your best to reduce your salt intake.

Aneurysm

The increase of blood pressure will make your blood vessels to bulge and weakened, which leads to forming "aneurysm." It can be life-threatening, if an aneurysm ruptures.

Not adding much potassium to your diet.

It is the potassium that aids the balance of the amount of sodium, in your cells. In a situation, that you don't retain enough potassium or you don't get enough potassium in your diet, it will lead to, too much accumulation of sodium in your blood and this can lead to high blood pressure. Consider potassium when preparing your next meal.

Some severe (chronic) conditions

Kidney disease, sleep apnea, and diabetes, which are all chronic conditions, can lead to the increase of your blood pressure.

Also, one of the conditions that can contribute to high blood pressure is pregnancy.

Note: Children may also be at risk of high blood pressure, even though, it is mostly common with adults. Some of the determinants, when it comes to children having high blood pressure, are heart and kidney problems. When they have these two conditions, they are likely to get high blood pressure. In the same vein, lack of exercise, unhealthy diet, and obesity which are all poor lifestyle habits, can also contribute to high blood pressure in children.

Complications that may come up because of Hypertension

Your blood vessel can get damaged due to the excessive pressure on your artery walls caused by high blood pressure, and also the organs in your body are not left out. If your blood pressure gets higher, and if it is not controlled, then it will cause more damage.

Below are the complications that will come up due to uncontrolled high blood pressure:

Difficulty in understanding and trouble with memory

If the high blood pressure you're experiencing is not controlled, it may affect your ability to learn, remember, and think. Most of the people, who have issues with understanding and trouble with memory, are people with high blood pressure.

Metabolic syndrome

This syndrome is a compilation of disorders of your body's metabolism, which includes high triglycerides; increased waist circumference; the "good" cholesterol: high-density lipoprotein (HDL) cholesterol; high insulin levels and high blood pressure. You will easily develop stroke, diabetes, and heart disease with these conditions.

Narrowed and weakened vessels in your kidneys.

When the above occurs, it can prevent the organs from functioning normally.

Narrowed, thickened, or torn blood vessels in the eyes – this can result to loss of sight or vision.

Heart failure

In order to pump blood against the higher pressure in your vessels, it is expected of the heart to work harder. As a result, the walls of the heart's pumping chamber will be very thick (left ventricular hypertrophy). So, it will be hard for the thickened muscle to pump adequate blood, required by the body, which can lead to heart failure.

Stroke or heart attack

One of the effects of hypertension is the thickening and hardening of the arteries (atherosclerosis), and this may lead to getting stroke, a heart attack, and other complications.

CHAPTER TWO

HOW TO LOWER BLOOD PRESSURE

You may be scared, after seeing the above complications that comes into play, due to high blood pressure and mostly, you may be very frightened, because it can be life-threatening.

If you're battling with this parlous foe called high blood pressure, don't panic. They are ways to lower your blood pressure numbers and manage hypertension. Reading further, you'll come across easy and straightforward techniques and tips, to help you lower your blood pressure. Those things consist of what you can do daily, to cancel your risk of dying early. For you to get a stronger heart, to live longer, and have healthier blood vessels, you should endeavor to include the following tips into your daily living. Don't go a day, without practicing it. With it, you will live longer and you'll not die because of hypertension.

1. USE OLIVE OIL TO COVER SALADS

Vegetables such as carrots, lettuce, and cabbage, which are full of nitrites, are believed to make compounds called nitro fatty acids, when olive oil is being put on them according to a study. The reason why, this transformation do happen is that, olive oil contains unsaturated fats, and the enzymes which are created, will help to lower blood pressure. So, try and do this when consuming your fruits and see how your blood pressured will be lowered.

2. ENGAGE IN MEDITATION FOR TWO AND A HALF HOURS EVERY WEEK

The above should not be a new thing to you. It is popularly known that, practicing mindfulness and meditation, has been a wonderful source of stress-reliever, for a lot of people. It helps to lower your stress, and when it happens thus, it helps to reduce your blood pressure numbers. A study was conducted, and it shows that, engaging in mindfulness behaviors like yoga, sitting meditation, and body scans for two and half hours, can lower blood pressure by around 5 mmHg.

Even when you're very busy with work, you should find time to meditate. Whenever you meditate, your mind will be free from worry, anxiety, depression, and you'll experience calmness. They are a lot of benefit to derive from the act of meditating.

Extra tip: One of the ways to live longer is to be mindful. If you're mindful and meditate frequently, you'll not age quickly.

You can meditate during your leisure time at work or at home. Just find a serene environment and practice meditation.

3. SAY NO TO ARTIFICIAL SWEETS

You may think that, it is only added sugar, you should run from when trying to lower blood pressure and losing weight. But, it is also important to avoid any artificial sweeteners. A research was conducted and it shows that, sucralose and aspartame, which are fake sweeteners, are likely to increase your risk of developing high blood pressure.

Don't consume such sweeteners. If you're addicted to them, try and break free from that addiction. It may be very sweet but, it can do you more harm than good, so run from them.

A friend of mine used to say, "Anything that is too sweet, can kill." The saying is very true, because naturally, sugars and sweeteners are very pleasant to the mouth. But health wise, too much of it is very dangerous. Run away from anything that can affect your health, no matter how sweet it seems to be. Remember, it is when you're alive and healthy, that you can enjoy the things of this world, your health first before pleasure.

4. ENDEAVOR TO DRINK A CUP OF YOGURT EVERY MORNING

It was discovered through a study, that there's a beneficial bacteria which lives in our gut, that is capable of restricting the effects of high-salt diets, and in turn, helps to keep blood pressure normal. To keep our gut healthy, foods and yogurt that contain good bacteria, such as sauerkraut, kefir, and kimchi, should be considered. They are called probiotics.

Whenever, you wake up in the morning drink a cup of yogurt, it will help to reduce your blood pressure.

5. AT HOME, TRY TO CHECK YOUR BLOOD PRESSURE FREQUENTLY

To be on top of your health, you need to monitor it at home. Because if you do this, you'll be able to know the sickness you're suffering from, and possibly find solution or cure for it.   It is important to check your blood pressure level at home. Even if it is not all the time, endeavor to schedule some time to check your blood pressure at home. It will help you. A study was conducted by University of Oxford Scientists, they found that people who are living with hypertension, who checked themselves at home - and had treatment from doctors outside the home - were able to lower it by a significant 3.2mmHg compared to the sets of people, who relied solely on doctor's appointments.

6. GET YOURSELF A PET

It does not matter the kind of pet, it can be a bird, dog, or a reptile. Try and get yourself one. You'll be able to have fun and beat stress, when you have a pet. Multiple studies on this, shows that, there's tremendous benefits to be derived from the companionship and stress-reducing play time you get from a pet, in the area of lowering your blood pressure.

If you don't own a pet, get yourself a pet today. When you're playing with a pet, you'll likely forget all your worries which will help to reduce or lower your blood pressure. If you hate pets, for your own benefit start loving them today.

7. GO FOR TESTING FREQUENTLY

It is good to check yourself at home. However, you may not have the necessary equipment to do this. You may have to visit your doctor, grocery stores, or your local pharmacy to check or measure your blood pressure every week. If you're able to know your blood pressure number, you'll look for a way to lower it.

Don't be a procrastinator. Endeavor to check your blood pressure more often.

8. CONSIDER HAVING A CUP OF SWEET POTATOES

When you avoid taking too much salt, your blood pressure will be normal, also, in the same vein, it will be helpful, if you add potassium-packed foods. Your system will get more potassium, if you eat foods such as beans, spinach, avocados, and sweet potatoes. It has been shown to prompt the kidneys to expel more salt, according to a study.

9. CONSUME WATERMELON DAILY

It contains antioxidants, vitamins, fiber, and minerals that can give you a healthy and nourished body. Also, they contain arginine, and amino acids citrulline. A study was conducted on watermelon effects on blood pressure, in the year 2010 and it was discovered that, watermelon extract containing 6 grams of aminos was able to reduce blood pressure in adults that are healthy.

I'm sure, you like watermelon, take it each day and see how your blood pressure will be reduced.

10. YOU SHOULD NOT OVER WORK

If you're a type that can work tirelessly, then you need to reduce it. In life, we must work to earn, but when it is too much on us it may result to some serious complications or issues.

In the case that you're working under someone, you should inform him or her, that long and stressful days on the clock can make you feel sick. There was a study that took place and it shows that working three or more hours over a normal seven-hour a day may increase the risk of dying from heart-related complications or problems such as high blood pressure by 60%.

If you find yourself in such situation, as earlier stated, tell your boss about it, so that you guys can come to a compromise.

''Your health first before wealth.''

11. DRINK SOME HERBAL TEA

It was discovered, through a study that, drinking four cups of herbal tea, which contain some hibiscus every day, can aid the lowering of blood pressure. The researchers have the idea that the photochemical in the ingredient helps to reduce inflammation in the blood vessels.

Herbal tea will help you to lower your blood pressure, so start taking it regularly, or at least twice a week.

12. IMPROVE YOUR SEXUAL LIFE

When you have a nice and energetic sex, it can help you to drop some stress levels by releasing endorphins. This sensual stress-reduction technique will help in reducing your blood pressure. You will feel good after having sex. Try and have sex frequently, you can have sex at least five times a week. Sex plays a crucial role in lowering blood pressure.

13. ENDEAVOR TO TAKE IN A CUP OF BEET JUICE

Even though, it is not that tasty, drinking a glass of beetroot juice every day can help to reduce blood pressure, according to a research. The high levels of nitrates work to expand blood vessels, which in turn allow for easier passage and lower pressure.

14. CONSIDER TAKING A LOT OF HOT PEPPERS

They are active ingredients in hot peppers, and whenever you take it, your mouth will be hot, like it is been set on fire. Capsaicin is responsible for that. A research has shown that, fiery compound can aid the lowering of high blood pressure, because it enable the blood vessels to relax and make it easier for more blood to flow through.

15. EMBARK ON A WALKOUT EVERY HOUR

It was discovered that, a person's health will be improved, when he or she stands up and move around in the day time. A study also shows that, walking for at least 12 minutes after sitting for a while can make your blood vessels to open up and restore blood flow. When you sit down for 7-9 hours a day, the blood flow in your legs will be greatly reduced. If you like to sit down a lot, you should try and learn how to be walking around, because it will help you more than you can imagine.

16. ENDEAVOR TO SLEEP AT LEAST 48-MINUTE DURING THE DAY

You may be very busy, but it will be good, if you schedule some time during the day to sleep. If you can sleep at least 48-minute in the day, you'll increase your chance of lowering or reducing your blood pressure. A research was conducted on this issue in some years back, the research discovered that, 48 - and 60 minutes sleep in the daytime can help to reduce blood pressure readings by a significant amount. If you're finding it hard, to sleep in the daytime, you should consider a "coffee nap." It works perfectly.

17. TRY TO LIMIT YOUR USE OF SMART PHONE

Smart phones are very good and they make life very easy. You can do a lot of thing with your smart phone like; chatting, texting, facebook, streaming of songs, replying emails, and watching videos etc. However, the attention you give to doing all those things on your smart phone can increase your stress and also your blood pressure. Smartphone can be very addictive, but for your own good, you should set aside some time when you'll drop your phone without using it.

18. CONSIDER A SPINACH SALAD

Potassium helps to clear sodium from your body and that is what spinach is made of. It also contains plant compounds, which is able to reduce appetite and control the urge to consume salty foods which may leads to gaining of weight. A study in 2017 shows that, a high body mass index has been linked to high blood pressure.

19. ENDEAVOR TO LAUGH FREQUENTLY

If you learn how to be happy, relax, and laugh often, your health will be greatly improved. You'll also have a stronger cardiovascular system. Your brain will release dopamine and subsequently circulate a compound that reduces blood pressure, when you live a happier and more humorous life, according to a research.

Life can be hard at times, but you're responsible for your happiness. So, even when you're sad or depressed, you should laugh and smile in order to stop your blood pressure from going higher.

20. TRY TO LIFT WEIGHTS FOR AN HOUR EVERY WEEK

A recent study shows that, lifting weights for an hour a week can aid in lowering high blood pressure by 17%. Also, it will be good, if you can add some aerobic exercise, researchers note that – the mix was shown to be the most protective to the cardiovascular system.

21. DEVIATE FROM TAKING ENERGY DRINKS

People, who are in need of a boost, will likely consume some beverages, but those kinds of drinks can lead to high blood pressure, you need to stop taking them. Some of them contain a lot of taurine and caffeine, and both can affect heart function and blood pressure. This was discovered through some studies. If you like taking such drinks, or you drink them to boost energy, you need to stop it, for your own good.

22. CONSIDER TAKING A FISH OIL SUPPLEMENT

In cold-water fish like salmon and mackerel, omega-3 fatty acids are found, and they are very crucial when it comes to heart health. You may have to turn to a high-quality fish oil supplement, in order to get enough, to lower high blood pressure. According to a study, it shows that; most docs recommend up to 1,000mg a day.

23. EXPOSE YOURSELF TO SUNLIGHT FOR A WHILE

It is a well known fact that, when an individual sits in the sun, especially in the morning, he or she receives or get vitamin D. In the same vein, according to a study your blood pressure, will be lowered when you expose your skin to sunlight. The rays make levels of nitric oxide in the skin and blood to rise, which relaxes blood vessels and reduce blood pressure.

24. AVOID NOISY ENVIRONMENT

Whenever you want to sleep, it is very important to make your bedroom dark and cool. Aside that it is also important to live in a quiet environment. It was discovered through a study that, to have a restorative and restful sleep, even moderate loud noises—like a humming air conditioner is capable of raising your blood pressure. So, endeavor to turn off anything that can cause noise in your environment which is capable of disrupting your sleep, and raising your blood pressure.

24. EAT DARK CHOCOLATE

It was discovered, through a recent studies, that eating dark chocolate can reduce blood pressure in the people who are living with hypertension. Dark chocolate contains heart-healthy cocoa flavanols, or plants compounds, which helps to boost blood vessel functioning.

25. BLEND UP A BATCH OF GAZPACHO

The fresh veggies that go into making up a great bowl of gazpacho—olive oil, garlic, cucumber, and onions have all been shown to lower high blood pressure. But the combo amps up the effect and make the cold soup a killer hypertension tamer, according to a study in the year 2012.

26. ADD YOGA AND CARDIO TO YOUR WORKOUTS

Your workout routine will have the extra punch to reduce blood pressure, when you do some yoga and add cardio, according to a recent study. It was also found by researchers, that by combining the two (yoga and cardio), cholesterol and body mass can easily be reduced.

27. CONSIDER LEAN BEEF

Many diets which are suggested to reduce blood pressure, seems to leave out red meat entirely, however, a new research shows that, getting a lean cuts of beef each day has been shown to be heart-healthy. You should consider lean cuts like flap steak, round roast, and sirloin, and add enough veggies and fruits, too.

28. GO TO THE FOREST AND HAVE YOUR BATHE

I'm sure, you've heard about "the Japanese-invented act of forest-bathing, or shinrin-yoku. If you've not heard about it before, it is the act of going to the forest to take your bathe, it can help to limit production of stress hormones and also, reduce blood pressure. In order to experience its soothing benefits, you don't need to travel down to Japan, what you're expected to do, is to locate a local forest and take time and slowly enjoy the green space and the trees.

29. CONSIDER GETTING ON A ROWER

Are you afraid of running on a treadmill or despise the looking manic on the elliptical? If so, try taking a seat at the rower when it's time for some heart-pounding cardio. Rover can utilize more muscles with each motion, which entails that, enough blood moving through your body and stronger blood vessels, according to studies.

30. TRY TO REDUCE YOUR SNORING WHEN SLEEPING

It can be very irritating to people around you, when you're snoring. Apart from that, it shows that you're suffering from a sleeping disorder like sleep apnea. A single instance of sleep apnea disrupts the bodies attempt at regulating blood pressure, which can cause harm to blood vessels and contribute to heart disease.

Do everything possible to stop the habit of snoring.

31. ENDEAVOR TO SWEAT IN A SAUNA REGULARLY

It may seem a little counter-intuitive, but it was discovered that frequenting a sauna can reduce the risk of high blood pressure. Those who went on the research reported that people who went in the heat bath - four to seven times a week had a 50% lower blood pressure than those who only went once a week.

32. CONSIDER HIGH-FIBER FOODS

Chickpeas, black beans, pears, raspberries, are all foods high in fiber, and you should be consuming them every day. Due to the high fiber content in such foods, it helps to make us feel full for a long time, so we can more easily keep a healthy weight, and this is one of the key ways to keep blood pressure in check.

33. ENDEAVOR TO GET YOUR NECK ADJUSTED

Are you experiencing a pain in the neck, and also have blood pressure, it may be related to a misalignment of the C-1, or Atlas, vertebrae located high in the neck. There was a study and it shows that, an adjustment done by a chiropractor reduced blood pressure as much as taking two medications at once—and it lasted into the eighth week of the study.

34. SUPPLEMENT WITH WHEY PROTEIN

After lifting weight, it is a usual thing to slam down a shake made with protein powder; however, eating whey protein can help to combat high blood pressure. A study revealed that drinking low-cost protein beverages everyday can reduce pressure in those with hypertension.

35. CUT DOWN YOUR SODIUM INTAKE

You should not consume too much sodium; try to limit your sodium intake. Are you getting sodium more than the recommended quantity for a day (2, 300mg which is equivalent to one tsp) either from what is already from your meal or from added salt, if yes, limit it. When you consume too much salt, it can lead to disease of the heart, high blood pressure, and stiff arteries. Don't consume excess salt.

36. DRINK SOME TART CHERRY JUICE

As revealed by a study, it reported that drinking some tart Montmorency cherry juice can lower high blood pressure at a similar amount compared with taking medication. The drop, which was measured at 7mmHg lower in the three hours after drinking, is more than what's required to reduce risk of stroke by 38%.

37. DO DEADLIFTS

When you engage in exercises, doing multi-joint, or compound, it challenge your body to get enough blood flowing, which make your blood vessels to be more relaxed and a stronger heart. You can do lunges, moves squats, and pushups, nevertheless, if you are pressed for time, at least do dead lifts as they work about 90% of your muscles in one movement.

38. STIR-FRY SOME TOFU

Isoflavones which is also found in peanuts and green tea is a compound found in soy products like tofu and soy milk. According to a study, it can provide significant blood pressure lowering properties. They are known to work on lowering blood pressure by increasing the enzymes that make nitric oxide.

39. SNACK ON HANDFUL OF RAISINS

These dried up little grapes contain plant compounds called polyphenols, along with antioxidants, potassium, and fiber. When you consume some raisins each day, your blood pressure will be significantly lowered according to a study in the year 2012. In the same vein, it was discovered that grapes can lower blood pressure too, so if you don't like raisin, consider mixing some grapes in your diet.

THE APPROPRIATE TIME TO VISIT A MEDICAL PRACTITIONER

You're required to visit your doctor, to check your blood pressure from time to time.

If you're a bit confused of – when to visit your doctor, take note of the below helpful suggestion.

If you're 18 years of age, ask your medical practitioner for a blood pressure reading at least every two (2) years. In the same vein, if you're older or at age 40, or you're between the age bracket of 18 to 39 (here, you're more prone to high blood pressure), ask your medical practitioner for a blood pressure reading every year.

To know if there is any disparity, blood pressure should be checked in both arms.

You're recommended to use an appropriate-sized arm cuff.

If you're diagnosed with high blood pressure, or you've other risk factors for cardiovascular disease, your doctor may suggest more regular readings. As part of their yearly checkups, children who are between the age of 3 or 4, and older children will usually have their blood pressure measured.

In the case that, you're not opportune to see your doctor often, you should consider getting a free blood pressure screening at a health resource fair or other locations in your community. Also, in some stores, you can get access to machines which are capable of measuring your blood pressure, without paying a dime.

Even at that, some public blood pressure machines, like those ones seen in pharmacies, may provide helpful information about your blood pressure; however, they may have some limitations. For these machines to be accurate in dispensing the right information – they are some factors to be considered such as using the machine properly and making sure you're getting the correct cuff size. Before making use of public blood pressure machines, endeavor to ask your doctor to advice you on how to go about it.

CHAPTER THREE

RECIPES FOR HIGH BLOOD PRESSURE (30 DAYS)

Controlling hypertension or high blood pressure is not hard, and it can be fun with healthy recipes such as Walnut-Rosemary Crusted Salmon, Eggplant Parmesan, and Slow-Cooker Chicken Stew. Reading further, you'll come across some recipes in a 30-day dinner plan and it follows the principles of a healthy blood pressure diet (incorporating recommendations from both the American Heart Association and the DASH diet) to deliver flavorful recipes that include lean protein, heart-healthy fats, enough vegetables, high-fiber whole grains, to keep your blood pressure in check each day.

So, let's take a look at those recipes, starting from day 1.

One (1) of thirty (30)

Day one (1): Roasted Salmon with Greens and Smoky Chickpeas

In this healthy salmon dinner, you'll get a dose of greens and green dressing! Consuming more of dark leafy greens a week, can help keep your brain in top shape. This dish features the Test Kitchen's current go-to method for doctoring a can of chickpeas: spice them up and roast until crispy.

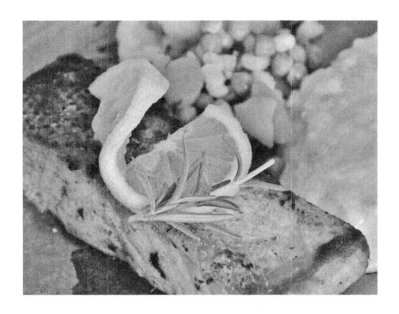

Two (2) of thirty (30)

Day two: Pesto Buddha and Charred Shrimp

Pesto Buddha and shrimp bowls are healthy, pretty, delicious, and it does not take too much time to get down. So, in essence they are most easy weeknight dinner. You can also add some vegetables and swap the shrimp for edamame, tofu, steak, or chicken.

Three (3) of thirty (30)

Day 3: Crispy Oven-Fried Fish Tacos

These fish tacos make a satisfying meal the whole family will cherish. In the restaurant, they are deep-fried, but what this book is going to show you, includes coating the fish in a seasoned whole-grain breading and sprinting it lightly with cooking spray before baking on a rack until golden brown. The result is a crispy exterior with moist and flaky fish inside.

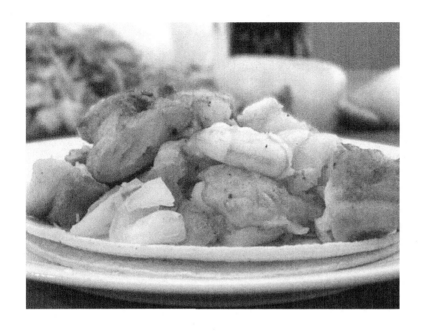

Four (4) of thirty (30)

Day 4: Potato Curry and Chickpea

This fast Indian-style curry comes together with ingredients that is readily available, like chickpeas, frozen peas, and canned tomatoes. In addition, making use of these spices reveals how easy it is to prepare a curry sauce for an easy vegetarian recipe.

Serve with whole-wheat naan to sop it all up.

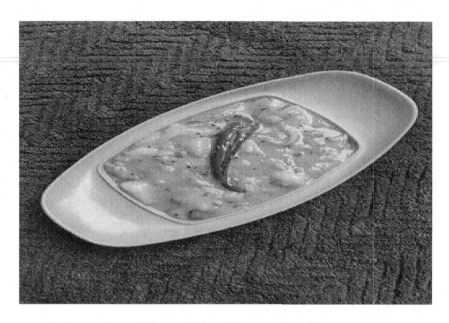

Five (5) of thirty (30)

Day 5: Bean Tostadas and Charred Vegetable with Lime Crema

Black beans and pile vegetables onto crisp tostadas and top them off with lime crema for a vegetarian dinner the entire family will love. Charring the vegetables under the broiler infuses them with smoky flavor while cooking them quickly.

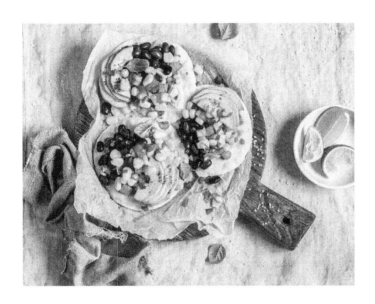

Six (6) of thirty (30)

Day 6: Southwest Salmon Chowder

It is good for a cold day; this salmon chowder is an ardent source of high quality omega-3 fatty acids and lean protein. It can be prepared in just some few minutes. It does not take time to prepare.

Day 7: Sheet-Pan Chicken Fajitas

One sheet pan is all you require to whip up these zesty chicken fajitas. They're easy and quick to make and cleanup is even faster!

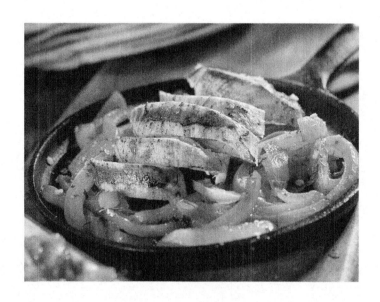

Eight (8) of thirty (30)

Day 8: White Bean Stew and Slow-Cooker Chicken

This load-and-go slow-cooker chicken recipe is good for a busy weeknight dinner. Serve this Tuscan-inspired dish with a glass of Chianti, a salad and crusty bread.

Day 9: Spaghetti with Quick Meat Sauce

You should consider this easy spaghetti with meat sauce on a midnight, rather than opening a jar of sauce. You should serve with garlic bread and steamed broccoli. The recipe makes enough for 8 servings. You should cook 8 ounces of spaghetti and freeze the leftover sauce, if you're serving only four for dinner.

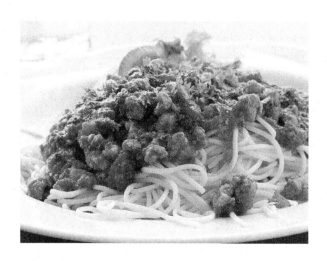

Ten (10) of thirty (30)

Day 10: Cucumber Lettuce Wraps with Peanut Sauce and Chicken

We love the crunch from sliced cucumber and jicama in these savory chicken lettuce wraps. Serve with the simple peanut sauce for an easy dinner recipe that will impress both adults and kids.

Eleven (11) of thirty (30)

Day 11: Creamy Lemon Pasta with Shrimp

You can consider using yogurt as substitute for cream in the sauce for this easy pasta recipe. What you need to do, is to warm the yogurt (you're not to boil it) and add some pasta-cooking water to thin it out. Fresh basil and lemon brighten up the whole-wheat pasta and complement the shrimp in this quick dinner recipe.

Day 12: Maple-Spice Carrots with Pumpkin Seed Salmon

At times, you may spend a lot of time, being busy at work – thereby coming to your house at late hours. The above can be prepared in just 35 minutes, so you may have to consider it. Maple-spiced carrots cook alongside pepita-crusted salmon fillets and deliver amazing taste and nutrition in a dinner the entire family will enjoy.

Day 13: Roasted Root Vegetables with Polenta and Goat Cheese

The above is a very healthy food – a bowl of creamy, soft polenta topped with warm roasted vegetables infused with sage and garlic.

Day 14: Eggplant Parmesan

This lighter take on eggplant parmesan maintains all the flavors of the classic dish but instead of frying, it is baked. There are also 11 grams of filling protein in this hearty vegetarian side dish.

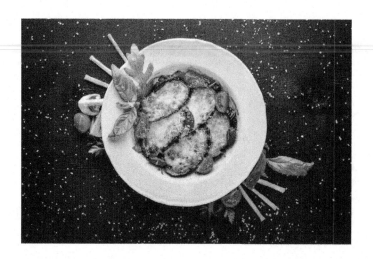

Fifteen (15) of thirty (30)

Day 15: Pan-Seared Steak with Crispy Herbs & Escarole

It takes just 20 minutes to get prepared, and it is easy to prepare. You may consider, preparing it at night after a busy day at work. Cooking herbs in the pan with the steak releases their aroma, infusing it into the meat while creating a crispy garnish. After the steaks and herbs are pan-seared, the escarole is cooked in the same skillet, therefore, this healthy dinner requires minimal cleanup too.

Sixteen (16) of thirty (30)

Day 16: Lemon Crusted Salmon and Coriander with Poached Eggs and Asparagus Salad

Lemon zest and crushed coriander seeds give this quick salmon recipe a nice flavor that pairs beautifully with poached egg salad and a shaved asparagus. When served with a glass of white wine, this healthy recipe makes the ultimate lunch or light dinner.

Seventeen (17) of thirty (30)

Day 17: Vegetable Penne and Chicken with Parsley-Walnut Pesto

The thought of preparing homemade pesto can make you feel nervous; nevertheless, in this quick pasta recipe you can make a simple sauce in a few minute, while the pasta water comes to a boil. Instead of fresh, you can consider frozen green beans and cauliflower. Cook the frozen vegetables according to package directions before tossing with the pesto and pasta.

Day 18: Vegan Roasted Vegetable Quinoa Bowl with Creamy Green Sauce

In a vegan riff on green goddess dressing, cashews provide a creamy base with tons of flavor from herbs and apple-cider vinegar. Drizzle it all over this bowl of quinoa and roasted vegetables to make a satisfying vegan dinner or easy packable lunch that is ready in just 30 minutes.

Nineteen (19) of thirty (30)

Day 19: Chicken Chili Verde

Prepared salsa verde adds tang to this fast weeknight chili recipe and pairs beautifully with creamy beans and the rich caramelized chicken. Consider poblano peppers, don't avoid them. Even though, the heat they offered, is not much. They can deliver a depth of flavor you'll not find in regular green bell peppers.

Twenty (20) of thirty (30)

Day 20: Peppery Barbecue-Glazed Shrimp with Orzo and Vegetables

In this healthy Barbecue shrimp recipe, shrimp are seasoned with a peppery spice blend and served with peppers, zucchini, and whole-grain orzo for a delicious and easy dinner. It can be prepared in just 30 minutes. The veggies and shrimp are cooked in the same skillet; therefore cleanup is a snap too.

Twenty one (21) of thirty (30)

Day 21: Tomato Pasta and Grilled Eggplant

It is awesome, when there is a slight combination of sweet tomatoes and smoky grilled eggplant. The eggplant-tomato mixture served over whole-wheat pasta with fresh basil and a bit of salty cheese makes an easy, healthy weeknight dinner.

Twenty two (22) of thirty (30)

Day 22: Broccoli and Sesame-Garlic Beef with Whole-Wheat Noodles

A savory marinade with sesame oil, soy sauce, garlic, and ginger infuses flavor into sirloin steak pieces in this healthy beef and broccoli stir-fry recipe. **Extra tip:** Partially freeze the beef for easier slicing.

Twenty three (23) of thirty (30)

Day 23: Super food Chopped Salad with Creamy Garlic Dressing and Salmon

Curly kale forms the base of this salad, but you could use spinach or chard. Add plenty of chopped veggies, like carrots, broccoli, and cabbage to the greens. Finish with rich salmon for protein and a drizzle of creamy yogurt dressing to bring it all together.

Twenty four (24) of thirty (30)

Day 24: Chinese Ginger Beef Stir-Fry with Baby Bok Choy

All of the ingredients for this easy beef stir-fry recipe are cooked in one wok (or skillet), so not only is the meal-prep fast for this healthy dinner, cleanup is quick too. In your grocery store, look for Lee Kum Kee Premium oyster-flavored sauce in the Asian-foods aisle. It has the most concentrated oyster flavor.

Twenty five (25) of thirty (30)

Day 25: No-Cook Black Bean Salad

When going on picnics, it will be nice to consider a classic black bean salad. It gets its creaminess from blended avocado. To give this hearty salad a peppery kick, you should try arugua, even though mixing of salad greens do work well.

Day 26: Pork Paprikash with Cauliflower "Rice"

Instead of regular rice, in this 30 minutes pork paprikash recipe, cut calories and carbs by using cauliflower "rice."

Day 27: Spicy and Sweet Roasted Salmon with Wild Rice Pilaf

Fresh jalapeños give this easy and quick roasted salmon dish its kick; balsamic and honey vinegar give it a sweet finish. A nutty-tasting wild rice pilaf completes this healthy dinner that comes together in some few minutes.

Twenty eight (28) of thirty (30)

Day 28: Pineapple Slaw and Jerk Chicken

This can be prepared in just 30 minutes; you may consider this spicy chicken dish with sweet pineapple slaw in any night of the week.

Twenty nine (29) of thirty (30)

Day 29: Green Chile Stew and Pork

Leave your slow cooker to do the work – while you're at work! - And come home to a delicious bowl of hearty stew for dinner. This filling stew recipe takes just 25 minutes to prepare in the morning, and it is full of chunks of pork sirloin, green chiles, hominy, and potatoes.

Thirty (30) of thirty (30)

Day 30: Chicken Curry Stuffed Sweet Potatoes

Make use of convenience ingredients, such as cooked chicken (purchased or leftover) and store-bought curry sauce to whip up these easy loaded baked potatoes. In this recipe, we are using cauliflower; however you can use any veggies you've at home for easy and quick dinner. Likewise, you can use sweet potatoes instead of russets.

Printed in Great Britain
by Amazon

23493038R00064